How to burn fat:

Rehabilitate your metabolism and live longer with the help of the foods you eat to enrich your diet.

By

Kathy M. Roush

Copyright © by Kathy M. Roush 2024. All rights reserved.

TABLE OF CONTENT

Introduction:

Burning fat is a sensitive process that involves lowering excess body weight by primarily targeting and metabolizing stored fat for energy. Fat burning is a complicated metabolic process that incorporates hormones, genetics, and lifestyle variables. It is necessary to generate a calorie deficit, wherein you consume fewer calories than your body requires, urging it to utilize fat stores for fuel. To understand how to burn fat properly, it's vital to investigate the science behind weight loss. The body stores energy in the form of fat and transforms it into usable fuel through a process called beta-oxidation. When you consume fewer calories than you spend, your body has little alternative but to draw into its fat reserves for energy, resulting in weight loss.

Here are some basic ways to help you burn fat effectively:

 Maintain a Balanced Diet: Consuming full, nutrient-dense meals like fruits, vegetables, lean proteins,and whole grains while eliminating processed foods and sugary snacks is vital. Whole foods are frequently more satisfying and healthy than processed foods, helping you sustain a calorie deficit without feeling deprived.

Incorporate Regular Exercise: Exercise is vital to burn excess calories and establish a calorie deficit. Engage in a combination of aerobic activities (such as jogging, cycling, or swimming) and strength training exercises to raise your metabolism and enhance fat burning. Strength training builds muscle, which boosts your resting metabolic rate, meaning you burn more calories even when at rest.

Stay Hydrated: Drinking an adequate amount of water not only promotes general health but also aids in the fat-burning process by maintaining proper metabolic activity. Water eliminates wastes from the body, promoting the breakdown of lipids and the outflow of poisons.

Get Sufficient Sleep: Adequate sleep is crucial to promote metabolism and hormonal balance, all of which are necessary for efficient fat loss. Aim for 7-9 hours of excellent sleep each night to manage hormones connected to hunger and metabolism, which might affect your body's capacity to burn fat efficiently.

Manage Stress: Chronic stress might impair weight loss efforts by encouraging the buildup of fat around the abdomen area. Stress causes the hormone cortisol, which boosts hunger and encourages the body to retain fat. Practice relaxation techniques such as meditation, deep breathing exercises, or yoga to reduce stress levels. This book contains simple tactics and advice for naturally burning fat and healing your metabolism. Sit back, relax, and stay tuned for these life-changing solutions.

Chapter 1

Things to be aware of about our health

The absence of disease or infirmity is not the only definition of health; rather, health is a condition of complete well-being on all levels, including the physical, the mental, and the social. When it comes to our health, the following information ought to be known.

Dietary Balance: A well-balanced diet is vital for overall health since it supplies the key nutrients that are required for the operations of the body.

Hydration: Maintaining proper hydration is critical for a variety of biological activities, including digestion, circulation, and the regulation of temperature.

Exercise regularly: Physical activity is essential for keeping a healthy weight, maintaining cardiovascular health, and sustaining overall well-being.

Getting Enough Sleep: Getting enough quality sleep is essential for maintaining cognitive function, bolstering the immune system, and maintaining general mental and physical health.The importance of mental health cannot be overstated; mental well-being is on par with physical health. Effective stress management and mindfulness practices are examples of useful practices.

Checkups on a Regular Basis: Having regular checkups can assist in the early detection of potential problems, which in turn increases the likelihood that treatment will be successful.

Vaccinations: Vaccines protect against preventable diseases, contributing to individual and societal health.

Avoiding Smoking: Smoking is a big risk factor for several health conditions, including lung cancer and cardiovascular disease.

Limiting Alcohol Consumption: Excessive alcohol intake can lead to liver damage, cardiovascular troubles, and other health problems.

Sun Protection: Protecting the skin from damaging UV radiation helps prevent skin cancer and premature aging.

Regular Dental Care: Oral health is linked to overall health. Regular dental check-ups and oral hygiene practices are vital.

Eye Care: Regular eye exams help maintain healthy eyesight and discover any eye issues early.

Hand Hygiene: Proper handwashing minimizes the risk of infections and the transmission of illnesses.

Posture Awareness: Maintaining proper posture helps prevent musculoskeletal disorders and increases overall comfort.

Stress Reduction: Chronic stress can significantly damage both physical and mental health, so finding effective stress-reduction measures is vital.

Healthy Relationships: Positive social ties contribute to emotional well-being and general health.

Limiting Processed Foods: A diet high in processed foods can contribute to obesity, heart disease, and other health difficulties.

- **Portion Control:** Controlling portion sizes helps maintain a healthy weight and aids digestion.

Regular Cardiovascular Exercise: Activities like walking, running, or cycling promote heart health and boost overall fitness.

Strength exercise: Building muscle through resistance exercise helps support metabolism and overall strength.

Flexibility Exercises: Stretching and flexibility exercises promote joint health and reduce the chance of injuries.

Mind-Body Connection: Practices like yoga and meditation strengthen the mind-body connection, boosting general well-being.

Breathing Exercises: Deep breathing exercises help relieve stress, improve lung function, and boost relaxation.

Bone Health: Adequate calcium and vitamin D diet, coupled with weight-bearing workouts, enhance bone health.

Regular Screenings: Depending on age and gender, screenings for illnesses including cancer, diabetes, and cholesterol levels are important.

Immune System Support: A healthy lifestyle, including good nutrition and frequent exercise, supports a powerful immune system.

Allergies: Understanding and treating allergies is vital for avoiding allergic responses.

Balanced Hormones: Hormonal balance is crucial for different biological activities, and hormonal imbalances can damage health.

Cholesterol Levels: Monitoring and regulating cholesterol levels are critical for cardiovascular health.

Blood Pressure: Regular blood pressure readings help identify and control hypertension.

Regular Detoxification: The body naturally detoxifies, however encouraging this process through healthy habits might be advantageous.

Posture at Work: Maintaining correct ergonomics at work helps prevent concerns like back pain and repetitive strain injuries.

Caffeine Intake: Moderating caffeine usage aids improved sleep and general health.

Avoiding Self-Medication: Consulting healthcare specialists before self-medicating is vital to prevent potential problems.

Understanding Family Medical History: Knowing family medical history assists in detecting genetic predispositions and adopting preventive actions.

Healthy Fats: Including sources of healthy fats, such as avocados and almonds, is vital for general health.

Fiber Intake: Adequate fiber ingestion supports digestive health and helps prevent constipation.

Blood Sugar Management: Monitoring and managing blood sugar levels are critical, especially for those with diabetes.

Proper Footwear: Wearing appropriate footwear helps foot health and prevents disorders like plantar fasciitis.

Adequate Iron Intake: Iron is important for carrying oxygen in the blood, and a lack can lead to anemia.

Brain Health: Mental stimulation, social interaction, and a good diet contribute to brain health.

Alcohol and Medication Interactions: Some medications may interact poorly with alcohol, so it's vital to be aware of potential hazards.

Sexual Health: Regular check-ups and safe habits contribute to overall sexual health.

Regular Vaccinations: In addition to childhood vaccinations, adults may need booster doses or extra vaccines.

Importance of Laughter: Laughter has great impacts on mental health and helps alleviate stress.

Environmental Health: Being conscious of environmental elements, such as air and water quality, can impact overall health.

Mindful Eating: Paying attention to eating patterns helps reduce overeating and supports good digestion.

Joint Health: Maintaining joint health through good nutrition and exercise is vital for mobility.

Understanding Medication Side Effects: Being aware of the potential side effects of drugs is vital for educated healthcare decisions.

Regular Learning: Keeping the mind engaged through continual learning adds to cognitive health and overall well-being.

Chapter 2

The Surprising Science of Fat, Health & Disease

It is vital to recognize that fat, or adipose tissue, which is largely formed of many individual fat cells (adipocytes) is not intrinsically bad. On the contrary, adipose tissue is vitally required to allow the body to store excess calories during periods when we ingest more calories than we expend through activity and resting metabolism. By doing so, adipose tissue works as a buffer of surplus calories, and so protects other tissues of the body from storing fat (i.e. heart, liver, muscle). This viewpoint is best demonstrated by the fact that persons who completely lack fat tissue (a disorder known as congenital lipodystrophy) are exceedingly unhealthy and are practically sure to acquire diabetes and heart disease, despite having an athletic and lean appearance.

In other words, fat tissue is vital for health. Where many people get into problems is when they have exhausted their body's ability to store extra calories in adipose tissue — we all have a specific threshold beyond which our fat depots can expand. When we get to that stage, our fat cells get so enormous that they are no longer able to buffer excess calories and hence cannot protect other tissues from fat accumulation and harm. This is when many of the basic metabolic problems of obesity become apparent - higher blood lipids, blood glucose levels, etc.

But wait, isn't losing fat through diet and exercise excellent for health?

Yes, whether we expend more energy (exercise) limit the amount of food we eat (diet) or both, our body draws on our additional stores of energy in our adipose tissue – this process eventually reduces the size of the individual fat cells. That is, fat loss happens due to a reduction in the size of fat cells, not a drop in the number of fat cells. Not unexpectedly, your jeans start fitting better. Also, this process makes fat cells more efficient at sucking up excess calories the next time we again eat more than we spend.

What about liposuction?

Fat reduction by diet/exercise is fundamentally different from the scenario of liposuction, where a big bunch of fat cells is removed from the body - that is, you reduce the number of fat cells, but the remaining ones don't grow any smaller or healthier. In reality, the opposite may be true, with less area to store excess calories than before surgery, hence the growth of those fat cells left behind. In a 2004 study, obese women who underwent abdominal liposuction, losing approximately 30- 45 % of the subcutaneous fat in the abdominal region (~10kg of fat), did not show improvements in any of the metabolic markers assessed, including insulin sensitivity, blood pressure, blood glucose, insulin, or lipid levels. Just to recap: merely surgically eliminating subcutaneous fat tissue does not make one healthier.

The truth about fats the good, the bad, and the in-between

Avoid trans fats, minimize saturated fats, and replace them with vital polyunsaturated fats

Why are trans fats dangerous for you

polyunsaturated and monounsaturated fats beneficial for you, and saturated fats somewhere in between? For years, fat was a four-letter word. We were instructed to banish it from our diets whenever feasible. We shifted to low-fat foods. But the adjustment didn't make us healthier, possibly because we cut back on beneficial fats as well as detrimental ones.

You may question if it isn't fat bad for you, yet your body requires some fat from eating. It's a key source of energy. It helps you absorb some vitamins and minerals. Fat is needed to construct cell membranes, the crucial exterior of each cell, and the sheaths enclosing neurons. It is vital for blood coagulation, muscle action, and inflammation. For long-term health, some fats are better than others. Good fats include monounsaturated and polyunsaturated fats. Bad ones include industrial-made trans fats. Saturated fats fall somewhere in the center.

All fats have a similar chemical structure

A chain of carbon atoms connected to hydrogen atoms. What makes one fat distinct from another is the length and shape of the carbon chain and the number of hydrogen atoms attached to the carbon atoms. Seemingly modest changes in structure result in substantial differences in form and function.

Bad trans fats

The worst sort of dietary fat is the kind known as trans fat. It is a result of a process called hydrogenation that is used to transform good oils into solids and to prevent them from going rancid. Trans fats have no proven health advantages and there is no safe level of ingestion.

Eating foods rich in trans fats raises the amount of bad LDL cholesterol in the bloodstream and reduces the amount of healthy HDL cholesterol. Trans fats generate inflammation, which is connected to heart disease, stroke, diabetes, and other chronic illnesses. They contribute to insulin resistance, which increases the chance of developing type 2 diabetes. Even small levels of trans fats can affect health: for every 2% of calories from trans fat taken daily, the risk of heart disease doubles by 23%.

In-between saturated fats

Saturated fats are common in the American diet. They are solid at room temperature – think cold bacon grease, but what is saturated fat? Common sources of saturated fat include red meat, whole milk, and other whole-milk dairy meals, cheese, coconut oil, and many commercially produced baked goods and other foods.

The word "saturated" here refers to the number of hydrogen atoms around each carbon atom. The chain of carbon atoms retains as many hydrogen atoms as possible - it's saturated with hydrogens.

Is saturated fat unhealthy for you? A diet heavy in saturated fats can drive up total cholesterol, and tip the balance toward more unhealthy LDL cholesterol, which promotes blockages to form in arteries in the heart and elsewhere in the body. For that reason, most nutrition experts advocate reducing saturated fat to under 10% of calories a day.

A few of recent investigations have blurred the link between saturated fat and heart disease. One meta-analysis of 21 research found that there was not enough evidence to indicate that saturated fat raises the risk of heart disease, but that replacing saturated fat with polyunsaturated fat may indeed reduce the risk of heart disease.

Two other major studies narrowed the prescription slightly, concluding that replacing saturated fat with polyunsaturated fats like vegetable oils or high-fiber carbohydrates is the best bet for reducing the risk of heart disease but replacing saturated fat with highly processed carbohydrates could do the opposite.

Good monounsaturated and polyunsaturated fats

Good fats come mostly from veggies, nuts, seeds, and fish. They vary from saturated fats by having fewer hydrogen atoms linked to their carbon chains. Healthy fats are liquid at normal temperature, not solid. There are two primary kinds of healthy fats: monounsaturated and polyunsaturated fats.

Monounsaturated fats: When you dip your bread in olive oil in an Italian restaurant, you're getting largely monounsaturated fat. Monounsaturated lipids have a single carbon-to-carbon double bond. The result is that it has two fewer hydrogen atoms than saturated fat and a bend at the double bond. This structure keeps monounsaturated fats liquid at normal temperature.

Good sources of monounsaturated fats are olive oil, peanut oil, canola oil, avocados, and most nuts, as well as high-oleic safflower and sunflower oils.

The revelation that monounsaturated fat could be beneficial came from the Seven Countries Study during the 1960s. It indicated that people in Greece and other parts of the Mediterranean region enjoyed a low rate of heart disease despite a high-fat diet. The predominant fat in their diet, though, was not the saturated animal fat found in countries with higher incidence of heart disease. It was olive oil, which includes mostly monounsaturated fat. This finding generated a surge of interest in olive oil and the "Mediterranean diet," a way of eating regarded as a healthier choice today.

Although there's no suggested daily consumption of monounsaturated fats, the National Academy of Medicine advocates using them as much as possible combined with polyunsaturated fats to replace saturated and trans fats.

Polyunsaturated fats. When you pour liquid cooking oil into a skillet, there's a good possibility you're using polyunsaturated fat. Corn oil, sunflower oil, and safflower oil are common examples. Polyunsaturated fats are important fats. That means they're essential for normal body functions, but your body can't create them. So, you must receive them from food. Polyunsaturated fats are used to create cell membranes and the coating of neurons. They are needed for blood clotting, muscular action, and inflammation. A polyunsaturated fat has two or more double bonds in its carbon chain. There are two main forms of polyunsaturated fats: omega-3 fatty acids and omega-6 fatty acids. The numbers correspond to the distance between the beginning of the carbon chain and the first double bond. Both varieties give health benefits. Eating polyunsaturated fats in place of saturated fats or highly processed carbs reduces dangerous LDL cholesterol and improves the lipid profile. It also reduces triglycerides. Good sources of omega-3 fatty acids include fatty fish such as salmon, mackerel, sardines, flaxseeds, walnuts, canola oil, and un-hydrogenated soybean oil. Foods rich in linoleic acid and other omega-6 fatty acids include vegetable oils such as safflower, soybean, sunflower, walnuts, and corn oils.

Chapter 3

Heal your metabolism (How to burn fat)

What is metabolism?

We normally conceive of "metabolism" in terms of speed: the pace at which we change food into energy. Metabolism is described as the multiple chemical reactions — occurring at the same time – that take place in the body to transform food into energy.

Your metabolism relies on three factors:

Basal/Resting Metabolic Rate (BMR/RMR): About 60 percent of your entire metabolism is determined by your BMR/RMR, the rate at which you burn energy/calories to sustain vital biological activities including breathing, circulation, and your brain and organ function. Genetics, age, body composition, food, and illnesses like hypothyroidism also affect your BMR/RMR.

Active Energy Expenditure (AEE): About 25 percent of your metabolism is determined by your AEE, which includes both planned exercise and Non-Exercise Activity Thermogenesis, commonly known as NEAT. NEAT describes the reflexive, involuntary, and non-exercise motions you make throughout the day, i.e., fidgeting, jiggling your foot, standing, walking around, and maintaining excellent posture.

Thermic Effect of Food (TEF): About 15 percent of your metabolism is determined by the thermic effect of the food you eat. The thermic effect is the energy necessary to break down food and transform it into energy. Protein requires roughly 20 to 30 percent of its calories for conversion; carbs and lipids require around 5 to 15 percent.

What are the signs and symptoms of a slowed-down metabolism?

The most obvious indicators of a damaged, slow metabolism include weight gain, weight loss plateaus, and difficulty reducing weight – even on a low-calorie diet with exercise. Many other indications and symptoms of a sluggish metabolism match those of hypothyroidism. These include constipation, chronic weariness, brain fog, irritability, mood changes, unpredictable or nonexistent menstrual cycles, muscle loss, low immunity against infection, and sleep difficulties. In addition, some persons with a slow metabolism have digestive problems such as feelings of excessive hunger, heartburn, gas, acid reflux, bloating, and diarrhea.

Some of the risk factors for a sluggish metabolism include:

- One or more episodes of fast weight loss ("crash diets")

- A history of weight loss followed by a recovery of weight (yo-yo dieting)

- A diagnosis of hypothyroidism

- A prior eating disorder

How does crash dieting or yo-yo dieting induce weight gain and reduce your metabolic rate?

Crash dieting triggers the body to go into famine mode. Your body protects itself by becoming incredibly effective at absorbing more calories from food. At the same time, your body also purposefully conserves stored energy and consumes less of it. It's a double whammy that results in a slower metabolism. When you crash diet, other systems are triggered that make it more likely your metabolism will stall, and you'll regain the weight. For example, with decreasing energy intake, physical activity levels normally drop.

Crash dieting also negatively affects your thyroid function. Specifically, it decreases T3 levels, can develop or aggravate hypothyroidism, and further restricts your metabolism. Other hormones are also altered by sudden weight loss. During and after crash dieting, the stress hormone cortisol increases, producing inflammation, lowering your metabolism, and making your body more

successful at accumulating fat. Rapid weight reduction can also trigger a leptin dip, -- the hormone that helps you feel full -- or make you resistant to leptin. When you have low leptin or leptin resistance, you feel hungry and are prone to eat more. Crash dieting can also raise ghrelin levels, the hunger hormone, making you feel hungrier.

Ultimately, that a crash diet decreases your metabolism significantly more than slower weight loss, and, following a crash diet, your metabolism stays sluggish, often for years…even if you regain the weight.

How can you heal a malfunctioning metabolism after crash diets and yo-yo dieting?

The tendency for the metabolism to stay low after a crash diet and cause rebound weight gain sometimes leads to weight cycling, or what is known as "yo-yo dieting." When you're yo-yo dieting, you establish a calorie deficit and lose weight swiftly, followed by a reduction in your metabolic rate. You'll notice that it's easier to regain weight, even after lowering daily calories. You recover the weight, and with a reduced metabolic rate, you'll need to reduce calorie intake even more to lose weight gain. It's a terrible loop!

To break the cycle, you need to focus on practical ways you can help raise the pace of your metabolism and restore it to a healthier state. Here are some of the greatest techniques to get your metabolism back on track.

Optimize your thyroid function

Because crash and yo-yo dieting can produce hypothyroidism, a complete thyroid evaluation is vital to your metabolic health. This can reveal a previously undiagnosed case of hypothyroidism or indicate the less-than-optimal treatment for your current hypothyroidism. It's helpful to start with a thyroid blood test panel. Ensure the panel includes Thyroid Stimulating Hormone (TSH) and Free T4, Free T3, and Thyroid Peroxidase (TPO) Antibodies. The results will help you understand how your thyroid functions and if it may negatively affect your metabolism. If you are hypothyroid, you'll need to work with a skilled doctor to optimize your thyroid hormone replacement treatment to support a healthy metabolism and weight loss.

Eat a healthful, nutrient-dense, gut-friendly diet

After a crash diet or yo-yo diet cycle, you must focus on eating the healthiest, most nutrient-dense diet you can. This involves choosing organic, pesticide-free, natural foods as much as possible and avoiding processed foods. Your emphasis should be on fruits and vegetables, healthy fats, nutritious proteins (such as fish and grass-fed meats), and anti-inflammatory fermented foods.

You should also pay attention to your intestinal health. A healthy stomach can more efficiently absorb and store food, burn energy as needed, and eliminate waste. You may also wish to integrate more spicy foods into your everyday diet. Capsaicin, a vital component found in several hot foods like peppers, has been demonstrated to increase metabolism.

Increase your protein intake

Many experts agree that increasing your protein can help your metabolism. You burn more calories when you eat protein compared to carbohydrates or fat. Protein also helps you grow muscle, which helps improve your metabolic level.

Various experts advocate eating at least 1 gram of protein per pound of body weight every day to support your metabolism.

Increase your fiber intake

Increasing your fiber intake can help raise metabolism since fiber requires more energy to digest, process, and remove. Aim for roughly 25 grams a day of fiber from foods and fiber supplements. Fiber supplements might help you meet the goal of 25 grams per day.

Eat the majority of your food early in the day

When you eat also has an impact on your metabolism. Most experts believe that eating a protein-rich breakfast helps boost and maintain metabolism and improve fat-burning throughout the day. You may also consider making dinner your lightest meal of the day. You can also fast from evening until breakfast. This helps you maintain healthier leptin levels and gives your body time to utilize stored energy for your nocturnal energy demands.

Stay well hydrated

You'll want to ensure you routinely drink water throughout the day. Drinking 2 liters of water every day boosts energy expenditure by roughly 100 calories daily. For an extra push, make it cold water; it stimulates metabolism a bit more than water at room temperature.

Drink coffee and tea

Caffeine can assist in enhancing metabolism. I illustrate that roughly 100 milligrams of caffeine – what you'd ordinarily get in a modest cup of coffee – might enhance your BMR/RMR by about 3 to 4 percent. Several servings of coffee at intervals throughout the day can enhance metabolism by as much as 11 percent. Moderation is important, however. Going overboard on coffee might worsen insulin resistance and blood glucose levels.

There's also scientific evidence that various teas – including black, green, oolong, and goji – can somewhat enhance your metabolism and fat burning. Tea also delivers increased hydration, which can significantly you in weight loss.

Use exercise and strength training to enhance muscle mass

The best activity you can do to assist in enhancing your metabolism is growing muscle. Increasing your muscle mass with activities like lifting weights, resistance machines, or Pilates will boost your Basal/Resting Metabolic Rate. Strength exercise can also assist in protecting your metabolism following a low-calorie diet. I observed that when following a low-calorie diet, women who undertook resistance training could lose weight without a change in metabolism compared to women who did either aerobic or no activity at all.

Increase your activity level...carefully

Many metabolism specialists recommend avoiding extended periods of vigorous aerobic activity since it elevates cortisol levels. Elevated cortisol wreaks havoc on your metabolism, boosting insulin and glucose levels and decreasing your metabolism.

If you wish to conduct aerobic exercise, shorter intervals of intensity – i.e., high-intensity interval training (HIIT) –

give many benefits of aerobic exercise with less danger of elevating cortisol.

You can also enhance your metabolism by raising your NEAT. As a beginning point, it can be good to incorporate regular periods of standing and walking throughout the day.

Get adequate sleep

Getting enough sleep is vital for your metabolism. Experts advise that 7 to 9 hours per night should be your target. "Short sleep" of less than 7 hours contributes to a vast variety of hormonal alterations, including blood sugar and cortisol rises. Short sleep diminishes the satiety hormone leptin levels, increases the hunger hormone ghrelin, and raises your risk of insulin resistance. I observed that just five days of short sleep led to a rise in food intake, leading to weight gain. Short sleep also affects your capacity to lose fat. Note that dieters who received only 5.5 hours of sleep during two weeks lowered their fat reduction by 55 percent!

Manage your stress

Active stress management is a vital aspect of altering a slow metabolism. Unmanaged stress boosts cortisol levels, negatively influencing glucose, insulin, and metabolism. Specifically, chronically high cortisol levels enhance belly fat storage, contributing to insulin resistance and weight gain.

The key to stress management is committing at least 10 minutes every day to your stress-reducing activity. What you do to handle stress depends on what approaches work best for you. Meditation, breath work, moderate yoga, tai chi, playing a musical instrument, or needlework are all valid stress-reducing activities. (Note: regular stress management is also helpful for your thyroid and immunological health!)

Breathe thoughtfully

The practice of mindfulbreathwork has two important metabolic benefits. First, diaphragmatic breathing is a natural stress reduction; a few calm, deep belly breaths can reduce cortical levels. Specific breathing techniques have also been tested and proven to assist in boosting

metabolism. Yoga activities such as left, right, or alternate nostril breathing can enhance oxygen intake and raise metabolism by as much as 37 percent.

Advice

Fixing a sluggish metabolism in part depends on having appropriate thyroid function. The Paloma Complete Thyroid Blood Test kit can get you started with easy and economical thyroid testing. Your at-home thyroid test kit has everything you need to collect and test your Thyroid Stimulating Hormone (TSH), Free T4, Free T3, and Thyroid Peroxidase (TPO) antibodies. You'll also have the opportunity to add on reverse T3 and vitamin D testing. New and seasoned hypothyroidism patients can then book a virtual visit with one of Paloma's top thyroid experts to discuss lab findings and decide the best treatment approach to restore normal thyroid function.

5 Ways to burn fat naturally

Burning fats naturally entails a combination of lifestyle decisions, including diet and exercise. Here are five strategies to help your body burn fat naturally:

1. Regular Exercise: Engage in regular physical activity to enhance your metabolism and promote fat burning. Cardiovascular exercises such as jogging, cycling, and swimming are helpful for burning calories. Additionally, incorporating strength training workouts helps build muscle, which in turn boosts your metabolic rate, even at rest.

2. Healthy Diet: Adopt a balanced and healthy diet that contains entire foods, such as fruits, vegetables, lean proteins, and whole grains. Focus on portion management and avoid excessive consumption of processed foods, sugary drinks, and high-calorie snacks. Include healthy fats, such as those from avocados, almonds, and olive oil, in moderation.

3. Hydration: Drink an adequate amount of water throughout the day. Staying hydrated is vital for several biological activities, including metabolism. Some research suggests that drinking water before meals may aid with weight loss by generating a sensation of fullness and reducing calorie consumption.

4. Adequate Sleep: Ensure you receive enough quality sleep each night. Lack of sleep can disturb hormonal

balance, leading to an increase in hunger hormones and a decrease in hormones that regulate satiety. Aim for 7-9 hours of sleep per night to improve overall health and metabolism.

5. Interval Training: Incorporate high-intensity interval training (HIIT) into your workout program. HIIT incorporates short bursts of intensive exercise followed by brief intervals of rest or lower-intensity activity. This sort of training has been demonstrated to be effective in burning fat and improving general fitness.

It's vital to note that spot reduction (losing fat from a specific location of the body) is not generally effective. Instead, focus on general fat loss through a mix of these lifestyle adjustments.

Chapter 4

Eating the Mediterranean way

What is the Mediterranean Diet?

The Mediterranean Diet is a manner of eating that emphasizes plant-based foods and healthy fats.

In general, if you follow a Mediterranean Diet, you'll eat:

- Lots of vegetables, fruit, beans, lentils and nuts.

- Lots of whole grains, such as whole-wheat bread and brown rice.

- Plenty of extra virgin olive oil (EVOO) as a source of healthful fat.

- A modest amount of fish, especially fish rich in omega-3 fatty acids.

- A reasonable amount of cheese and yogurt.

- Little or no meat, selecting chicken instead of red meat.

- Little or no sweets, sugary drinks, or butter.

- A modest amount of wine with meals (but if you don't currently drink, don't start).

A nutritionist can help you alter this diet as needed based on your medical history, underlying diseases, sensitivities, and preferences.

What is the definition of the Mediterranean Diet?

There are various definitions of the diet (each with slightly different aims for servings). That's because the diet focuses on overall eating patterns rather than specific formulas or computations. It's also based on dietary trends throughout several different Mediterranean countries, each with its unique quirks. Because there's no standard definition, the Mediterranean Diet is adaptable, and you can tailor it to your needs.

What are the benefits of the Mediterranean Diet?

The Mediterranean Diet offers many benefits, including Lowering your risk of cardiovascular disease.

- Supporting a body weight that's beneficial for you.

- Supporting healthy blood sugar, blood pressure, and cholesterol.

- Lowering your risk of metabolic syndrome.

- Supporting a healthy balance of gut microbiota (bacteria and other microbes) in your digestive tract.

- Lowering your risk for certain types of cancer.

- Slowing the decrease of brain function as you age.

- Helping you live longer.

Cardiologists commonly prescribe the Mediterranean Diet because significant evidence supports its heart-healthy effects. One study (published in 2018)

looked at people at high risk of cardiovascular disease during a five-year period. These people were split into two groups. One group followed the Mediterranean Diet, whereas the other group followed a low-fat diet. The Mediterranean Diet group showed a 30% decreased relative risk of cardiovascular events compared to the low-fat diet group. Such incidents included heart attack, stroke, or cardiovascular-related mortality.

Why is the Mediterranean Diet helpful for me?

The Mediterranean Diet comprises several different nutrients that work together to aid your health. There's no single item or ingredient accountable for the Mediterranean Diet's benefits. Instead, the diet is excellent for you because of the combination of nutrients it delivers.

Think of a choir with numerous members singing. One voice alone could carry part of the music, but you need all the voices to come together to produce the entire effect. Similarly, the Mediterranean Diet works by offering you a perfect balance of nutrients that harmonize to promote your health.

A Mediterranean Diet is excellent for you because it:

Limits saturated fat and trans fat. You need some saturated fat, but only in modest amounts. Eating too much-saturated fat might boost your LDL (bad) cholesterol. A high LDL boosts the risk of plaque accumulation in your arteries (atherosclerosis). Trans fat has no health benefits. Both of these "unhealthy fats" can promote inflammation.

Encourages healthful unsaturated fats, especially omega-3 fatty acids: Unsaturated fats boost healthy cholesterol levels, enhance brain health, and prevent inflammation. Plus, a diet strong in unsaturated fats and low in saturated fat maintains good blood sugar levels.

Limits sodium: A diet heavy in salt can elevate your blood pressure, placing you at greater risk for a heart attack or stroke.

Limits refined carbs, especially sugar: Foods heavy in refined carbs might cause your blood sugar to increase. Refined carbs also provide you with additional calories without much nutritious value. For example, such foods often have little or no fiber.

Favor foods strong in fiber and antioxidants: These nutrients help lower inflammation throughout your body. Fiber also helps keep waste flowing through your big intestine. Antioxidants defend you against cancer by warding off free radicals.

What does the Mediterranean Diet look like?

The Mediterranean Diet doesn't look the same for everyone. In general, it comprises an abundance of nutritious grains, vegetables, and fruit coupled with moderate portions of fish, legumes, and nuts.

How do I start a Mediterranean Diet?

You may have numerous questions as you begin a new food plan. It's vital to talk with a primary care physician or nutritionist before making major changes to your diet or starting any new eating plan. They'll make sure your planned plan is best for you based on your unique demands. They'll also provide meal plans and recipes for you to try at home.

As you get started, you might ask how much you can adjust the Mediterranean Diet without losing its benefits. Remember that the Mediterranean Diet is a general approach to eating. It's not a rigid diet with hard and fast guidelines. As a result, you can customize it to meet your needs (preferably with a dietitian's advice).Below are answers to some frequent queries you might have about adjustments.

Can the Mediterranean Diet be vegetarian?

Yes. If you want a vegetarian diet, you can easily adjust the Mediterranean Diet to omit meat and fish. In that situation, you'd acquire your protein completely from plant sources like nuts and beans. Talk to a dietitian to learn more.

Can the Mediterranean Diet be gluten-free?

Yes. You can adapt recipes to exclude gluten-based items. Talk to a dietician for recipe ideas and support in making any modifications.

Can I use normal olive oil instead of extra virgin olive oil?

Regular olive oil is a wonderful option for oil that's heavy in saturated fat (like palm oil). However, to receive the best benefits, opt for extra virgin olive oil.

A vital truth to know before starting the Mediterranean Diet is that not all olive oils are the same. The Mediterranean Diet demands for extra virgin olive oil (EVOO), specifically. That's because it has a healthy fat ratio. This means EVOO has more beneficial fat (unsaturated) than unhealthy fat (saturated). Aside from its fat ratio, EVOO is healthful since it's abundant in antioxidants.

Antioxidants help protect your heart and prevent inflammation throughout your body. Because it's made differently, normal olive oil doesn't contain these antioxidants.

Can I eat pizza on the Mediterranean Diet?

It depends on how you prepare it. Many American-style pizzas are heavy in sodium, saturated fat, and calories. These qualities make it less than optimal for fulfilling your Mediterranean Diet aims. Instead of eating out, try making your own heart-healthy pizza to gain more nutritional advantages.

Can I eat dishes from non-Mediterranean cultures?

The Mediterranean Diet describes dietary trends in one specific area of the world. That doesn't imply you should exclude dishes and recipes from different cultural traditions. It's crucial to design an eating plan that's beneficial for you physically, mentally, and socially. The Mediterranean Diet offers a style of eating that research ties to various health benefits. This diet focuses on typical patterns of eating. It doesn't ask you to study every single dietary choice or exclude specific foods. So, there's an opportunity to customize the Mediterranean Diet to your preferences and cultural traditions. This can mean keeping some traditional recipes the same (no ingredient substitutions) and eating them only on rare occasions. certain recipes might be just as good and special to you with certain modifications (such as olive oil instead of butter, or more herbs instead of salt). Working with a dietician might help you decide when and how to make replacements or other changes to your significant meals.

How does lifestyle relate to the Mediterranean Diet?

- To gain the most from your eating plan, strive to: Exercise often, ideally with others.

- Avoid smoking or using any tobacco products.

- Prepare and enjoy meals with family and friends.

- Cook more often than you dine out.

- Eat locally sourced foods whenever feasible.

When was the Mediterranean Diet created?

The concept of the Mediterranean Diet emerged in the 1950s. That's when an American researcher named Ancel Keys initiated the Seven Countries Study. This study spanned decades. It studied correlations between diet and cardiovascular disease over the world. As part of the study, Keys and his team looked into eating patterns in Greece and Italy in the 1950s and 1960s. They discovered those eating patterns were connected with decreased rates of coronary artery disease (compared with eating patterns in the U.S. and Northern Europe). Thus, the heart-healthy Mediterranean Diet was developed.

So, if you follow a Mediterranean Diet now, you're eating like people did in specific Mediterranean countries in the mid-20th century. Research demonstrates those trends have evolved over the years and no longer hold true in many Mediterranean countries.

There are visual pyramids and other instructions that teach you how to put a Mediterranean Diet into practice. A dietitian can help you review such resources and explain how to use them in your daily life.

NOTE

In a world with many diet options, it can be hard to decide which one is ideal for you. Research has demonstrated the benefits of the Mediterranean Diet for many people, especially those at risk for heart disease. Beyond protecting your heart, the Mediterranean Diet can help you prevent or treat many other conditions.

Chapter 5

Eat to beat protocol

Burning fat with diet entails making mindful choices about the things you eat and building a sustainable and balanced eating plan. Here are some ways to help you burn fat through your diet:

1. Caloric Deficit: The primary premise of fat reduction is sustaining a caloric deficit, which means ingesting fewer calories than your body requires to maintain its present weight. This can be achieved by either reducing calorie intake or increasing physical exercise.

2. Balanced Macronutrients: Ensure a balanced diet of macronutrients — carbs, proteins, and fats. Each macronutrient plays a key role in your body's processes, and a healthy ratio can help fat loss while keeping muscle mass.

3. Protein Intake: As said earlier Include a suitable amount of protein in your diet. Protein helps in keeping lean muscle mass, improves metabolism, and promotes satiety, helping you feel full for longer durations.

4. Healthy Fats: Choose healthy fats, such as avocados, nuts, seeds, and olive oil. These fats supply necessary nutrients and contribute to a feeling of fullness, which can help decrease overall calorie consumption.

5. Complex Carbohydrates: Opt for complex carbohydrates including whole grains, veggies, and legumes. They give prolonged energy and fiber, providing a sensation of fullness and reducing overeating.

6. Limit Added Sugars: Minimize the consumption of added sugars and refined carbohydrates. These can lead to rises in blood sugar levels and contribute to fat storage.

7. Hydration: Stay well-hydrated. Sometimes, the body can confuse thirst with hunger. Drinking water before meals may help you consume less calories.

8. Meal Timing: Consider smaller, more frequent meals throughout the day to balance blood sugar levels and control appetite. However, individual preferences and lives differ, so establish a mealtime schedule that suits you.

9. Limit Processed Foods: Processed foods generally contain hidden sugars, harmful fats, and empty calories. Choose full, nutrient-dense foods for better overall health and successful fat loss.

10. Regular Exercise: While this applies more to lifestyle than nutrition, adding regular physical activity can greatly contribute to fat burning. A combination of cardiovascular activities and strength training can be very useful.

Final summary: Unlocking your potential

Embarking on a path to battle stubborn diet-borne fat and restore your metabolism can be tough, but with the appropriate strategy, it is absolutely attainable. By adopting a holistic and sustainable strategy that incorporates healthy eating habits, regular exercise, stress management, and sufficient sleep, you may alter your body and improve your overall well-being.

Understand your body: Begin by analyzing your body's particular needs, including your metabolic rate, body composition, and nutritional requirements. Consult with a healthcare expert or a qualified dietician to acquire insights into your individual needs and goals.

Focus on balanced nutrition: Emphasize entire, nutrient-rich foods such as fruits, vegetables, lean meats, whole grains, and healthy fats. Avoid crash diets or excessive limits, as they might negatively affect your metabolism in the long run. Strive for a balanced approach and portion control.

Prioritize regular exercise: Incorporate both cardiovascular activities and strength training into your program. Cardio exercises like jogging, swimming, or cycling can help burn calories, while strength training builds muscle and enhances metabolism. Aim for at least 150 minutes of moderate-intensity aerobic activity per week, along with two or more strength training sessions.

Manage stress levels: Chronic stress can contribute to weight gain and metabolic disorders. Find healthy strategies to manage stress, such as practicing mindfulness, meditation, yoga, or indulging in hobbies that provide joy and relaxation. Prioritizing self-care might have a good impact on your metabolism.

Get adequate sleep: Sleep deprivation can affect your metabolism, leading to weight gain and increased hunger. Aim for 7-9 hours of decent sleep each night. Establish a consistent sleep regimen and establish a sleep-friendly environment to boost the quality of your rest.

Stay hydrated: Drinking an adequate amount of water not only helps with digestion but also improves your metabolism. Aim to drink at least 8 cups (64 ounces) of water every day, adjusting based on your activity levels.

Monitor progress and adjust as needed: Keep track of your progress by frequently evaluating your body composition, weight, and other important variables. Celebrate your achievements, and if required, make adjustments to your diet and exercise plan to keep working towards your goals.

How to burn fat